A Beginner Guide to Your Ketogenic Air Fryer Meals

A Handful of Quick, Delicious Recipes for Your Ketogenic Air Fryer Recipes

Morgan Parry

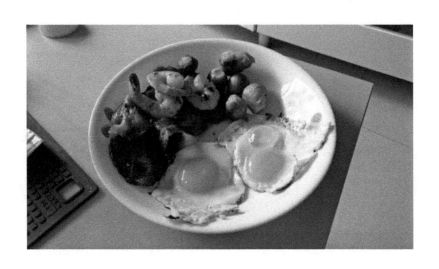

advice. The content within this book has been derived from various sources. Please consult a licensed professional before attempting any techniques outlined in this book.

By reading this document, the reader agrees that under no circumstances is the author responsible for any losses, direct or indirect, which are incurred as a result of the use of information contained within this document, including, but not limited to, — errors, omissions, or inaccuracies.

Table of Contents

Cumin Garlic 9

Brownies 10

Keto Butter Balls..13

Avocado Chocolate Brownies 16

Cardamom Bombs..18

Cream Cups...20

Butter Custard...21

Lemon Peppermint Bars...23

Avocado Cream Pudding...26

Chocolate Candies...28

Berry Pudding 30

Almond Bars..32

Creamy Sausage Bites...33

Shrimp Dip..35

Stuffed Eggs..37

Tuna Bowls..40

Lemon Tofu Cubes 42

Avocado Wedges 44

Sage Radish Chips...47

Bacon Dip..48

Eggplant Sticks..50

Crab Dip..52

Coconut Chicken Wings..54

Chicken and Berries Bowls...56

Chicken Wraps 59

Tomato Salad...60

Turmeric Cauliflower Popcorn...63

Tomato and Eggplant Casserole..66

Meatloaf...68

Beef and Sauce...70

Rosemary Olives Mix...73

Garlic Balsamic Tomatoes...75

Almond Eggplant Meatballs..76

Cilantro Broccoli Mix...79

Mustard Cabbage...80

Cajun Zucchini and Broccoli..82

Lime Olives and Zucchini...84

Cream Cheese Green Beans..85

Tomato Artichokes Mix..88

Sprouts Wraps..89

Cheese Zucchini Chips...91

Chocolate Bacon Bites...93

Almond Coconut Granola...94

Pickled Bacon Bowls..96

Tomato Smokies...97

Coconut Chicken Bites...99

Pizza Bites...101

Mozzarella Snack..104

Mushroom Pizza Bites..105

Cumin Garlic

Prep time: 5 minutes

Prep time: 10 minutes

Servings: 4

Ingredients:

- 2 garlic bulbs
- ½ teaspoon cumin seeds
- 1 teaspoon olive oil

Directions:

1.   In the shallow bowl mix up cumin seeds and olive oil. Then brush the garlic bulbs with oil mixture and put them in the air fryer. Cook the garlic for 10 minutes at 375F.

Nutrition: calories 18, fat 1.2, fiber 0, carbs 1.6, protein 0.1

Brownies

Preparation time: 10 minutes

Prep time: 25 minutes

Servings: 6

Ingredients:

- 6 tablespoons cream cheese, soft 3 eggs, whisked
- tablespoons cocoa powder
- tablespoons coconut oil, melted
- ¼ cup almond flour
- ¼ cup coconut flour
- ¼ teaspoon baking soda 1 teaspoon vanilla extract
- ½ cup almond milk
- 3 tablespoons swerve Cooking spray

Directions:

1. Grease a cake pan that fits the air fryer with the cooking spray. In a bowl, mix rest of the ingredients, whisk well and pour into the pan. Put the pan in your air

fryer, cook at 370 degrees F for 25 minutes, cool the brownies down, slice and serve.

Nutrition: calories 182, fat 12, fiber 2, carbs 4, protein 6

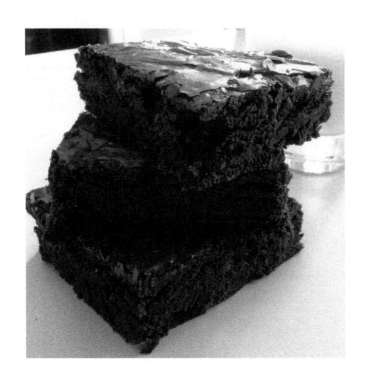

Keto Butter Balls

Prep time: 15 minutes

Prep time: 10 minutes

Servings: 4

Ingredients:

- 1 tablespoon butter, softened1 tablespoon Erythritol
- ½ teaspoon ground cinnamon
- 1 tablespoon coconut flour
- 1 teaspoon coconut flakes
- Cooking spray

Directions:

1. Put the butter, Erythritol, ground cinnamon, coconut flour, and coconut flakes. Then stir the mixture with the help of the fork until homogenous. Make 4 balls. Preheat the air fryer to 375F. Spray the air fryer basket with cooking spray and place the balls inside. Cook the dessert for 10 minutes.

Nutrition: calories 43, fat 3.3, fiber 1.3, carbs 2.9, protein 0.6

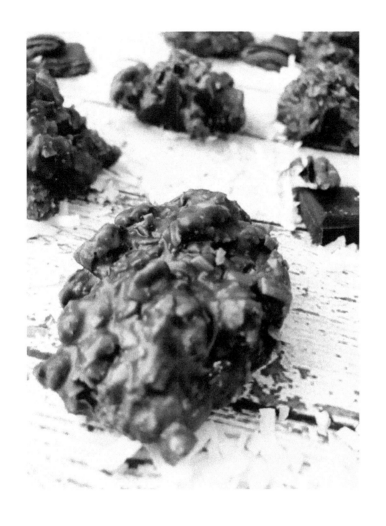

Avocado Chocolate Brownies

Preparation time: 10 minutes

Prep time: 30 minutes

Servings: 12

Ingredients:

- 1 cup avocado, peeled and mashed

- ½ teaspoon vanilla extract

- 4 tablespoons cocoa powder

- 3 tablespoons coconut oil, melted 2 eggs, whisked

- ½ cup dark chocolate, unsweetened and melted

- ¾ cup almond flour

- teaspoon baking powder

- ¼ teaspoon baking soda 1 teaspoon stevia

Directions:

1.   In a bowl, mix the flour with stevia, baking powder and soda and stir. Add the rest of the ingredients gradually, whisk and pour into a cake pan that fits the air

fryer after you lined it with parchment paper. Put the pan in your air fryer and cook at 350 degrees F for 30 minutes. Cut into squares and serve cold.

Nutrition: calories 155, fat 6, fiber 2, carbs 6, protein 4

Cardamom Bombs

Prep time: 10 minutes

Prep time: 5 minutes

Servings: 2

Ingredients:

- 2 oz avocado, peeled
- 1 egg, beaten
- ½ teaspoon ground cardamom
- 1 tablespoon Erythritol
- 2 tablespoons coconut flour
- 1 teaspoon butter, softened

Directions:

1.   Put the avocado in the bowl and mash it with the help of the fork. Add egg and stir the mixture until it is smooth. Then add ground cardamom, Erythritol, and coconut flour. After this, add butter and stir the mixture well. Make the balls from the avocado mixture and press them gently.

2.   Then preheat the air fryer to 400F. Put the avocado bombs in the air fryer and cook them for 5 minutes.

Nutrition: calories 143, fat 10.9, fiber 5, carbs 7.5, protein 4.9

Cream Cups

Preparation time: 5 minutes

Prep time: 10 minutes

Servings: 6

Ingredients:

- tablespoons butter, melted 8 ounces cream cheese, soft
- tablespoons coconut, shredded and unsweetened 3 eggs
- tablespoons swerve

Directions:

1. In a bowl, mix all the ingredients and whisk really well. Divide into small ramekins, put them in the fryer and cook at 320 degrees F and bake for 10 minutes. Serve cold.

Nutrition: calories 164, fat 4, fiber 2, carbs 5, protein 5

Butter Custard

Prep time: 15 minutes

Prep time: 35 minutes

Servings: 2

Ingredients:

- ¼ cup heavy cream
- 1 tablespoon Erythritol
- 1 teaspoon coconut flour
- 3 egg yolks
- 1 teaspoon butter

Directions:

1.   Whip the heavy cream and them mix it up with Erythritol and coconut flour. Whisk the egg yolks and add them in the whipped cream mixture. Then grease 2 ramekins with butter and transfer the whipped cream mixture in the ramekins. Preheat the air fryer to 300F. Put the ramekins with custard in the air fryer and cook them for 35 minutes.

Nutrition: calories 155, fat 14.4, fiber 0.5, carbs 2.1, protein 4.6

Lemon Peppermint Bars

Prep time: 15 minutes

Prep time: 16 minutes

Servings: 8

Ingredients:

- 1 teaspoon peppermint

- 1 cup almond flour

- 1/3 cup peanut butter

- ½ teaspoon baking powder

- 1 teaspoon lemon juice

- ½ teaspoon orange zest, grated

Directions:

1.   In the bowl, mix up almond flour, peppermint, baking powder, and orange zest. Then add peanut butter and lemon juice. Knead the non-sticky dough. Cut the dough on 8 pieces and roll the balls. Press them gently to get the shape of the bars. Preheat the air fryer to 365F. Line the air fryer basket with baking paper. Put 4 cookies

in the air fryer in one layer. Cook them for 8 minutes. Remove the cooked bars from the air fryer. Repeat the same steps with uncooked bars.

Nutrition: calories 84, fat 7.2, fiber 1.1, carbs 3.1, protein 3.5

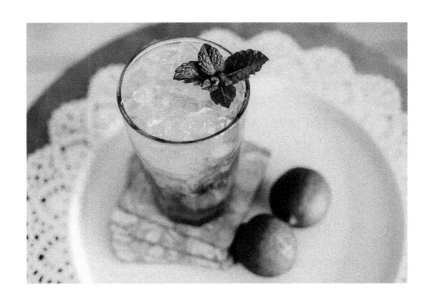

Avocado Cream Pudding

Preparation time: 5 minutes

Prep time: 25 minutes

Serving: 6

Ingredients:

- 4 small avocados, peeled, pitted and mashed 2 eggs, whisked
- 1 cup coconut milk
- ¾ cup swerve
- teaspoon cinnamon powder
- ½ teaspoon ginger powder

Directions:

1. In a bowl, mix all the ingredients and whisk well. Pour into a pudding mould, put it in the air fryer and cook at 350 degrees F for 25 minutes. Serve warm.

Nutrition: calories 192, fat 8, fiber 2, carbs 5, protein 4

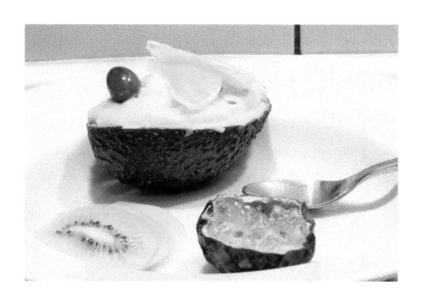

Chocolate Candies

Prep time: 15 minutes

Prep time: 2 minutes

Servings: 4

Ingredients:

- 1 oz almonds, crushed

- 1 oz dark chocolate

- 2 tablespoons peanut butter

- 2 tablespoons heavy cream

Directions:

1. Preheat the air fryer to 390F. Chop the dark chocolate and put it in the air fryer mold. Add peanut butter and heavy cream. Stir the mixture and transfer in the air fryer. Cook it for 2 minutes or until it starts to be melt. Then line the air tray with parchment. Put the crushed almonds on the tray in one layer. Then pour the cooked chocolate mixture over the almonds.

2. Flatten gently if needed and let it cool. Crack the cooked chocolate layer into the candies.

Nutrition: calories 154, fat 12.9, fiber 1.9, carbs 7.4, protein 3.9

Berry Pudding

Preparation time: 5 minutes

Prep time: 15 minutes

Servings: 6

Ingredients:

- cups coconut cream 1/3 cup blackberries 1/3 cup blueberries

- tablespoons swerve Zest of 1 lime, grated

Directions:

1. In a blender, combine all the ingredients and pulse well. Divide this into 6 small ramekins, put them in your air fryer and cook at 340 degrees F for 15 minutes. Serve cold.

Nutrition: calories 173, fat 3, fiber 1, carbs 4, protein 4

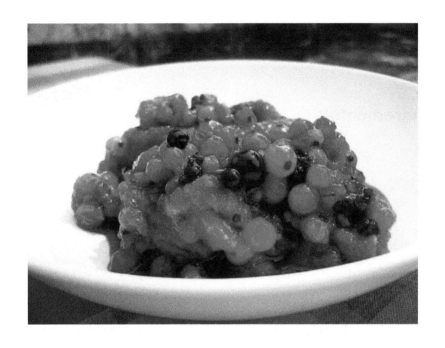

Almond Bars

Preparation time: 5 minutes

Prep time: 12 minutes

Servings: 12

Ingredients:

- teaspoon vanilla extract 1 cup almond butter, soft 1 egg

- tablespoons erythritol

Directions:

1. In a bowl, mix all the ingredients and whisk really well. Spread this on a baking sheet that fits the air fryer lined with parchment paper, introduce in the fryer and cook at 350 degrees F and bake for 12 minutes. Cool down, cut into bars and serve.

Nutrition: calories 130, fat 12, fiber 1, carbs 3, protein 5

Creamy Sausage Bites

Prep time: 10 minutes

Prep time: 9 minutes

Servings: 6

Ingredients:

- 1 cup ground pork sausages

- ¼ cup almond flour

- ¼ teaspoon baking powder

- ¼ teaspoon salt

- 1 teaspoon flax meal

- 1 egg, beaten

- ½ teaspoon dried dill

- 2 tablespoons heavy cream

- 1 teaspoon sunflower oil

Directions:

1. In the bowl mix up ground pork sausages, almond flour, baking powder, salt, flax meal, egg, dried dill, and

heavy cream. Make the small balls from the mixture. Preheat the air fryer to 400F. Place the sausage balls in the air fryer in one layer and cook them for 9 minutes. Flip the balls on another side after 5 minutes of cooking.

Nutrition: calories 67, fat 4.9, fiber 0.3, carbs 0.9, protein 5.4

Shrimp Dip

Preparation time: 5 minutes

Prep time: 20 minutes

 Servings: 4

Ingredients:

- 1 pound shrimp, peeled, deveined and minced 2 tablespoons ghee, melted

- ¼ pound mushrooms, minced

- ½ cup mozzarella, shredded 4 garlic cloves, minced

- 1 tablespoon parsley, chopped Salt and black pepper to the taste

Directions:

1.   In a bowl, mix all the ingredients, stir well, divide into small ramekins and place them in your air fryer's basket. Cook at 360 degrees F for 20 minutes and serve as a party dip.

Nutrition: calories 271, fat 15, fiber 3, carbs 4, protein 14

Stuffed Eggs

Prep time: 10 minutes

Prep time: 17 minutes

Servings: 4

Ingredients:

- 4 eggs
- 2 oz avocado, peeled, mashed
- 1 teaspoon lemon juice
- ¼ teaspoon butter, melted

Directions:

1. Place the eggs in the air fryer and cook them at 250F for 17 minutes. Then cool and peel the eggs. Cut the eggs into halves and remove the egg yolk. Churn the egg yolks with the help of the fork. Add butter, mashed avocado, and lemon juice. Stir the mixture until smooth. Fill the egg whites with the avocado mixture.

Nutrition: calories 94, fat 7.4, fiber 1, carbs 1.6, protein 5.8

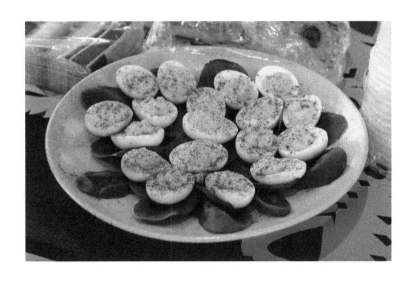

Tuna Bowls

Preparation time: 5 minutes

Prep time: 10 minutes

Servings: 2

Ingredients:

- 1 pound tuna, skinless, boneless and cubed 3 scallion stalks, minced

- 1 chili pepper, minced 2 tablespoon olive oil

- 1 tablespoon coconut cream 1 tablespoon coconut aminos 2 tomatoes, cubed

- 1 teaspoon sesame seeds

Directions:

1. In a pan that fits your air fryer, mix all the ingredients except the sesame seeds, toss, introduce in the fryer and cook at 360 degrees F for 10 minutes. Divide into bowls and serve as an appetizer with sesame seeds sprinkled on top.

Nutrition: calories 231, fat 18, fiber 3, carbs 4, protein 18

Lemon Tofu Cubes

Prep time: 10 minutes

Prep time: 7 minutes

Servings: 2

Ingredients:

- ½ teaspoon ground coriander
- 1 tablespoon avocado oil
- 1 teaspoon lemon juice
- ½ teaspoon chili flakes
- 6 oz tofu

Directions:

1. In the shallow bowl mix up ground coriander, avocado oil, lemon juice, and chili flakes. Chop the tofu into cubes and sprinkle with coriander mixture. Shake the tofu. After this, preheat the air fryer to 400F and put the tofu cubes in it. Cook the tofu for 4 minutes. Then flip the tofu on another side and cook for 3 minutes more.

Nutrition: calories 70, fat 4.5, fiber 1.1, carbs 1.9, protein 7.1

Avocado Wedges

Preparation time: 5 minutes

Prep time: 8 minutes

Servings: 4

Ingredients:

- 4 avocados, peeled, pitted and cut into wedges 1 egg, whisked

- and ½ cups almond meal

- A pinch of salt and black pepper Cooking spray

Directions:

1. Put the egg in a bowl, and the almond meal in another. Season avocado wedges with salt and pepper, coat them in egg and then in meal almond. Arrange the avocado bites in your air fryer's basket, grease them with cooking spray and cook at 400 degrees F for 8 minutes. Serve as a snack right away.

Nutrition: calories 200, fat 12, fiber 3, carbs 5, protein 16

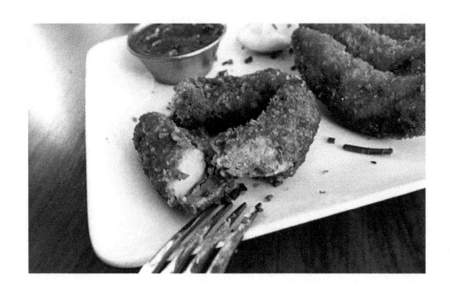

Sage Radish Chips

Prep time: 10 minutes

Prep time: 35 minutes

Servings: 6

Ingredients:

- 2 cups radish, sliced
- ½ teaspoon sage
- 2 teaspoons avocado oil
- ½ teaspoon salt

Directions:

1. In the mixing bowl mix up radish, sage, avocado oil, and salt. Preheat the air fryer to 320F. Put the sliced radish in the air fryer basket and cook it for 35 minutes. Shake the vegetables every 10 minutes.

Nutrition: calories 8, fat 0.3, fiber 0.7, carbs 1.4, protein 0.3

Bacon Dip

Preparation time: 5 minutes

Prep time: 20 minutes

Servings: 12

Ingredients:

- tablespoons ghee, melted

- cups spring onions, chopped A pinch of salt and black pepper

- 2 ounces cheddar cheese, shredded 1/3 cup coconut cream

- 6 bacon slices, cooked and crumbled

Directions:

1. Heat up a pan that fits the fryer with the ghee over medium-high heat, add the onions, stir and sauté for 7 minutes. Add the remaining ingredients, except the bacon and stir well. Sprinkle the bacon on top, introduce the pan in the machine and cook at and 380 degrees F

for 13 minutes. Divide into bowls and serve as a party dip.

Nutrition: calories 220, fat 12, fiber 2, carbs 4, protein 15

Eggplant Sticks

Prep time: 10 minutes

Prep time: 8 minutes

Servings: 3

Ingredients:

- 6 oz eggplant, trimmed
- ½ teaspoon dried oregano
- ½ teaspoon dried cilantro
- ½ teaspoon dried thyme
- ½ teaspoon ground cumin
- ½ teaspoon salt
- 1 tablespoon olive oil
- ¼ teaspoon garlic powder

Directions:

1. Cut the eggplant into the fries and sprinkle with dried oregano, cilantro, thyme, cumin, salt, and garlic powder. Then sprinkle the eggplant fries with olive oil and

shake well. Preheat the air fryer to 400F. Place the eggplant fries in the air fryer and cook them for 4 minutes from each side.

Nutrition: calories 58, fat 4.9, fiber 2.2, carbs 3.9, protein 0.7

Crab Dip

Preparation time: 5 minutes

Prep time: 20 minutes

Servings: 4

Ingredients:

- 8 ounces cream cheese, soft 1 tablespoon lemon juice

- 1 cup coconut cream

- 1 tablespoon lemon juice

- 1 bunch green onions, minced

- 1 pound artichoke hearts, drained and chopped 12 ounces jumbo crab meat

- A pinch of salt and black pepper

- 1 and ½ cups mozzarella, shredded

Directions:

1. In a bowl, combine all the ingredients except half of the cheese and whisk them really well. Transfer this to

a pan that fits your air fryer, introduce in the machine and cook at 400 degrees F for 15 minutes. Sprinkle the rest of the mozzarella on top and cook for 5 minutes more. Divide the mix into bowls and serve as a party dip.

Nutrition: calories 240, fat 8, fiber 2, carbs 4, protein 14

Coconut Chicken Wings

Prep time: 10 minutes

Prep time: 10 minutes

Servings: 4

Ingredients:

- 4 chicken wings

- 1 teaspoon keto tomato sauce

- 2 tablespoons coconut cream

- 1 teaspoon nut oil

- ¼ teaspoon salt

Directions:

1. Sprinkle the chicken wings with tomato sauce, nut oil, coconut cream, and salt. Massage the chicken wings with the help of the fingertips and put in the air fryer. Cook the chicken at 400f for 6 minutes. Then flip the wings on another side and cook for 4 minutes more.

Nutrition: calories 53, fat 4.6, fiber 0.2, carbs 0.7, protein 2.5

Chicken and Berries Bowls

Preparation time: 5 minutes

Prep time: 20 minutes

Servings: 2

Ingredients:

- 1 chicken breast, skinless, boneless and cut into strips 2 cups baby spinach

- 1 cup blueberries

- 6 strawberries, chopped

- ½ cup walnuts, chopped

- 3 tablespoons balsamic vinegar 1 tablespoon olive oil

- 3 tablespoons feta cheese, crumbled

Directions:

1. Heat up a pan that fits the air fryer with the oil over medium heat, add the meat and brown it for 5 minutes. Add the rest of the ingredients except the spinach, toss, introduce in the fryer and cook at 370 degrees F for 15

minutes. Add the spinach, toss, cook for another 5 minutes, divide into bowls and serve.

Nutrition: calories 240, fat 14, fiber 2, carbs 3, protein 12

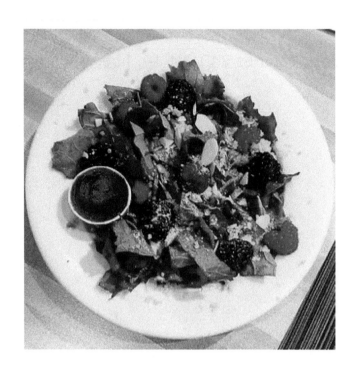

Chicken Wraps

Prep time: 10 minutes

Prep time: 10 minutes

Servings: 2

Ingredients:

- 6 oz chicken fillet
- 2 oz bacon, sliced
- 1 teaspoon avocado oil
- ¼ teaspoon ground black pepper

Directions:

1. Chop the chicken fillets into cubes and wrap in the bacon. Then slice the wrapped chicken nuggets with ground black pepper and avocado oil and place in the air fryer. Cook the nuggets for 10 minutes at 400F.

Nutrition: calories 319, fat 18.5, fiber 0.2, carbs 0.7, protein 35.2

Tomato Salad

Preparation time: 5 minutes

Prep time: 12 minutes

Servings: 6

Ingredients:

- 1 pound tomatoes, sliced

- 1 tablespoon balsamic vinegar 1 tablespoon ginger, grated

- ½ teaspoon coriander, ground 1 teaspoon sweet paprika

- 1 teaspoon chili powder

- 1 cup mozzarella, shredded

Directions:

1.   In a pan that fits your air fryer, mix all the ingredients except the mozzarella, toss, introduce the pan in the air fryer and cook at 360 degrees F for 12 minutes. Divide into bowls and serve cold as an appetizer with the mozzarella sprinkled all over.

Nutrition: calories 185, fat 8, fiber 2, carbs 4, protein 8

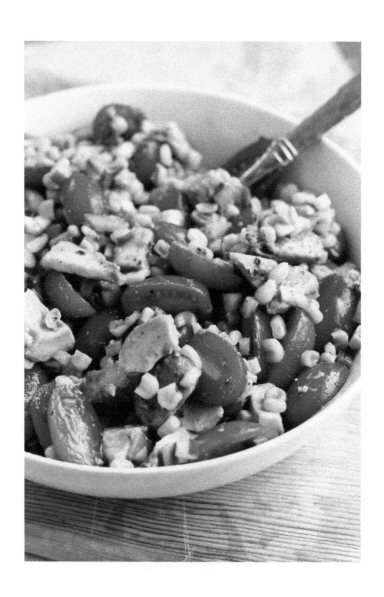

Turmeric Cauliflower Popcorn

Prep time: 10 minutes

Prep time: 11 minutes

Servings: 4

Ingredients:

- 1 cup cauliflower florets

- 1 teaspoon ground turmeric

- 2 eggs, beaten

- 2 tablespoons almond flour

- 1 teaspoon salt

- Cooking spray

Directions:

1.   Cut the cauliflower florets into small pieces and sprinkle with ground turmeric and salt. Then dip the vegetables in the eggs and coat in the almond flour. Preheat the air fryer to 400F. Place the cauliflower popcorn in the air fryer in one layer and cook for 7

minutes. Give a good shake to the vegetables and cook them for 4 minutes more.

Nutrition: calories 120, fat 9.3, fiber 2.3, carbs 4.9, protein 6.3

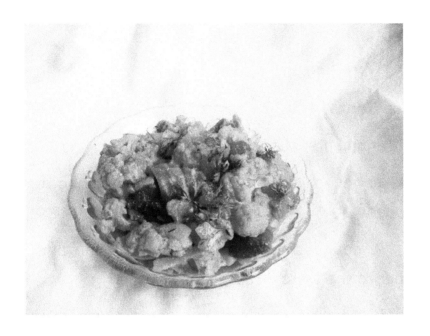

Tomato and Eggplant Casserole

Preparation time: 5 minutes

Prep time: 20 minutes

Servings: 4

Ingredients:

- eggplants, cubed

- 1 hot chili pepper, chopped 4 spring onions, chopped

- ½ pound cherry tomatoes, cubed Salt and black pepper to the taste 2 teaspoons olive oil

- ½ cup cilantro, chopped 4 garlic cloves, minced

Directions:

1. Grease a baking pan that fits the air fryer with the oil, and mix all the ingredients in the pan. Put the pan in the preheated air fryer and cook at 380 degrees F for 20 minutes, divide into bowls and serve for lunch.

Nutrition: calories 232, fat 12, fiber 3, carbs 5, protein 10

Meatloaf

Prep time: 10 minutes

Prep time: 20 minutes

Servings: 4

Ingredients:

- 2 cups ground beef
- 1 large egg, beaten
- 2 spring onions, chopped
- 1teaspoon garam masala
- ½ teaspoon ground ginger
- 1 teaspoon garlic powder
- ½ teaspoon salt
- ½ teaspoon ground turmeric
- ½ teaspoon cayenne pepper
- 1 teaspoon olive oil
- ¼ teaspoon ground nutmeg

Directions:

1.   In the mixing bowl mix up ground beef, egg, onion, garam masala, ground ginger, garlic powder, salt, ground turmeric, cayenne pepper, and ground nutmeg. Stir the mass with the help of the spoon until homogenous. Then brush the round air fryer pan with olive oil and place the ground beef mixture inside. Press the meatloaf gently. Place the pan with meatloaf in the air fryer and cook for 20 minutes at 365F.

Nutrition: calories 174, fat 10.8, fiber 0.8, carbs 3.7, protein 15.1

Beef and Sauce

Preparation time: 5 minutes

Prep time: 20 minutes

Servings: 4

Ingredients:

- 1 pound lean beef meat, cubed and browned 2 garlic cloves, minced

- Salt and black pepper to the taste cooking spray

- 16 ounces keto tomato sauce

Directions:

1. Preheat the Air Fryer at 400 degrees F, add the pan inside, grease it with cooking spray, add the meat and all the other ingredients, toss and cook for 20 minutes. Divide into bowls and serve for lunch.

Nutrition: calories 270, fat 15, fiber 3, carbs 6, protein 12

Parmesan Beef Mix

Preparation time: 5 minutes

Prep time: 20 minutes

Servings: 4

Ingredients:

- 14 ounces beef, cubed

- 7 ounces keto tomato sauce

- tablespoon chives, chopped

- tablespoons parmesan cheese, grated 1 tablespoon oregano, chopped

- 1 tablespoon olive oil

- Salt and black pepper to the taste

Directions:

1. Grease a pan that fits the air fryer with the oil and mix all the ingredients except the parmesan. Sprinkle the parmesan on top, put the pan in the machine and cook at 380 degrees F for 20 minutes. Divide between plates and serve for lunch.

Nutrition: calories 280, fat 14, fiber 4, carbs 6, protein 15

Rosemary Olives Mix

Preparation time: 5 minutes

Prep time: 15 minutes

Servings: 4

Ingredients:

- cups black olives, pitted and halved A handful basil, chopped

- 2 rosemary springs, chopped 2 red bell peppers, sliced

- 12 ounces tomatoes, chopped 4 garlic cloves, minced

- 2 tablespoons olive oil

Directions:

1. In a pan that fits the air fryer, combine the olives with the rest of the ingredients, toss, put the pan in the fryer and cook at 380 degrees F for 15 minutes. Divide between plates and serve.

Nutrition: calories 173, fat 6, fiber 2, carbs 4, protein 5

Garlic Balsamic Tomatoes

Preparation time: 5 minutes

Prep time: 15 minutes

Servings: 4

Ingredients:

- 1 tablespoon olive oil

- 1 pound cherry tomatoes, halved 1 tablespoon dill, chopped

- 6 garlic cloves, minced

- 1 tablespoon balsamic vinegar Salt and black pepper to the taste

Directions:

1. In a pan that fits the air fryer, combine all the ingredients, toss gently, put the pan in the air fryer and cook at 380 degrees F for 15 minutes. Divide between plates and serve.

Nutrition: calories 121, fat 3, fiber 2, carbs 4, protein 6

Almond Eggplant Meatballs

Prep time: 15 minutes

Prep time: 8 minutes

Servings: 7

Ingredients:

- 3 eggplants, peeled, boiled

- 1 egg, beaten

- 1 teaspoon minced garlic

- 3 spring onions, chopped

- ½ cup almond flour

- 1 teaspoon chives

- ½ teaspoon chili flakes

- ½ teaspoon salt

- 1 teaspoon sesame oil

Directions:

1.   Chop the boiled eggplants and squeeze the juice from them. After this, transfer the eggplants in the

blender. Add egg, minced garlic, spring onions, almond flour, chives, chili flakes, and salt. Grind the mixture until it is homogenous and smooth. After this, make the eggplant meatballs from the mixture with the help of the scooper. Preheat the air fryer to 380F. Put the eggplant meatballs in the air fryer and sprinkle them with sesame oil. Cook the meatballs for 8 minutes.

Nutrition: calories 87, fat 2.7, fiber 8.6, carbs 14.8, protein 3.6

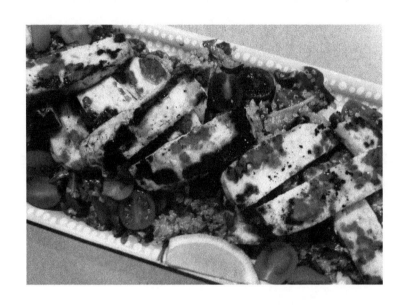

Cilantro Broccoli Mix

Preparation time: 5 minutes

Prep time: 15 minutes

Servings: 4

Ingredients:

- 1 broccoli head, florets separated 2 cups cherry tomatoes, quartered A pinch of salt and black pepper 1 tablespoon cilantro, chopped Juice of 1 lime

- A drizzle of olive oil

Directions:

1. In a pan that fits the air fryer, combine the broccoli with tomatoes and the rest of the ingredients except the cilantro, toss, put the pan in the air fryer and cook at 380 degrees F for 15 minutes. Divide between plates and serve with cilantro sprinkled on top.

Nutrition: calories 141, fat 3, fiber 2, carbs 4, protein 5

Mustard Cabbage

Prep time: 10 minutes

Prep time: 40 minutes

Servings: 4

Ingredients:

- 1-pound white cabbage
- 1 teaspoon mustard
- 1 teaspoon ground black pepper
- ½ teaspoon salt
- 3 tablespoons butter, melted
- ½ teaspoon ground paprika
- ½ teaspoon chili flakes
- 1 teaspoon dried thyme

Directions:

1.   In the mixing bowl mix up mustard, ground black pepper, salt, butter, ground paprika, chili flakes, and dried thyme. Brush the cabbage with the mustard

mixture generously and place it in the air fryer. Cook the cabbage for 40 minutes at 365F. Then cool the cooked vegetable to the room temperature and slice into Servings.

Nutrition: calories 111, fat 9.1, fiber 3.3, carbs 7.5, protein 1.9

Cajun Zucchini and Broccoli

Prep time: 10 minutes

Prep time: 15 minutes

Servings: 2

Ingredients:

- ½ zucchini, chopped

- 2 spring onions, chopped

- ¼ cup broccoli, chopped

- 1 teaspoon Cajun seasonings

- 1 teaspoon nut oil

- 2 oz fennel bulb, chopped

Directions:

1.   In the mixing bowl mix up all ingredients. Then preheat the air fryer to 385F. Put the mixture in the air fryer and cook it for 15 minutes. Shake the vegetables every 5 minutes.

Nutrition: calories 46, fat 2.5, fiber 2, carbs 5.8, protein 1.4

Lime Olives and Zucchini

Preparation time: 5 minutes

Prep time: 12 minutes

Servings: 4

Ingredients:

- 4 zucchinis, sliced

- cup kalamata olives, pitted Salt and black pepper to the taste 2 tablespoons lime juice

- tablespoons olive oil

- 2 teaspoons balsamic vinegar

Directions:

1. In a pan that fits your air fryer, mix the olives with all the other ingredients, toss, introduce in the fryer and cook at 390 degrees F for 12 minutes. Divide the mix between plates and serve.

Nutrition: calories 150, fat 4, fiber 2, carbs 4, protein 5

Cream Cheese Green Beans

Prep time: 15 minutes

Prep time: 5 minutes

Servings: 2

Ingredients:

- 8 oz green beans

- 1 egg, beaten

- 1 teaspoon cream cheese

- ¼ cup almond flour

- ¼ cup coconut flakes

- ½ teaspoon ground black pepper

- ½ teaspoon salt

- 1 teaspoon sesame oil

Directions:

1.   In the mixing bowl mix up cream cheese, egg, and ground black pepper. Add salt. In the separated bowl mix up coconut flakes and almond flour. Preheat the air fryer

to 400F. Dip the green beans in the egg mixture and then coat in the coconut flakes mixture. Repeat the step one more time and transfer the vegetables in the air fryer. Sprinkle them with sesame oil and cook for 5 minutes. Shake the vegetables after 2 minutes of cooking if you don't put green beans in one layer.

Nutrition: calories 149, fat 10.3, fiber 5.3, carbs 10.9, protein 6.1

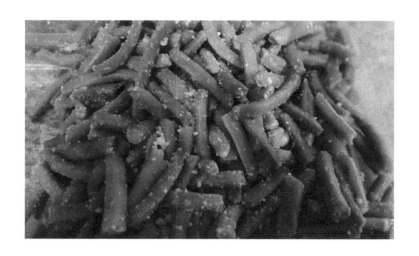

Tomato Artichokes Mix

Preparation time: 5 minutes

Prep time: 15 minutes

Servings: 4

Ingredients:

- 14 ounces artichoke hearts, drained 1 tablespoon olive oil
- 2 cups black olives, pitted 3 garlic cloves, minced
- ½ cup keto tomato sauce 1 teaspoon garlic powder

Directions:

In a pan that fits your air fryer, mix the olives with the artichokes and the other ingredients, toss, put the pan in the fryer and cook at 350 degrees F for 15 minutes. Divide the mix between plates and serve.

Nutrition: calories 180, fat 4, fiber 3, carbs 5, protein 6

Sprouts Wraps

Preparation time: 5 minutes

Prep time: 20 minutes

Servings: 12

Ingredients:

- 12 bacon strips
- 12 Brussels sprouts A drizzle of olive oil

Directions:

1. Wrap each Brussels sprouts in a bacon strip, brush them with some oil, put them in your air fryer's basket and cook at 350 degrees F for 20 minutes. Serve as an appetizer.

Nutrition: calories 140, fat 5, fiber 2, carbs 4, protein 4

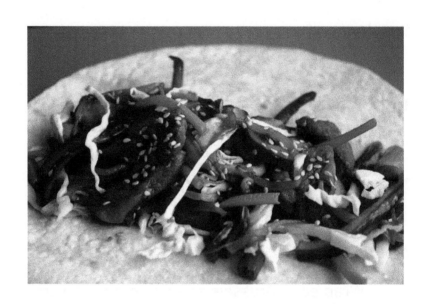

Cheese Zucchini Chips

Prep time: 10 minutes

Prep time: 13 minutes

Servings: 8

Ingredients:

- 2 zucchinis, thinly sliced

- 4 tablespoons almond flour

- 2 oz Parmesan

- 2 eggs, beaten

- ½ teaspoon white pepper

- Cooking spray

Directions:

1.   In the big bowl mix up almond flour, Parmesan, and white pepper. Then dip the zucchini slices in the egg and coat in the almond flour mixture.

2.   Preheat the air fryer to 355F. Place the prepared zucchini slices in the air fryer in one layer and cook them

for 10 minutes. Then flip the vegetables on another side and cook them for 3 minutes more or until crispy.

Nutrition: calories 127, fat 9.7, fiber 2.1, carbs 5.1, protein 7.3

Chocolate Bacon Bites

Preparation time: 5 minutes

Prep time: 10 minutes

Servings: 4

Ingredients:

- 4 bacon slices, halved

- 1 cup dark chocolate, melted A pinch of pink salt

Directions:

1. Dip each bacon slice in some chocolate, sprinkle pink salt over them, put them in your air fryer's basket and cook at 350 degrees F for 10 minutes. Serve as a snack.

Nutrition: calories 151, fat 4, fiber 2, carbs 4, protein 8

Almond Coconut Granola

Prep time: 10 minutes

Prep time: 12 minutes

Servings: 4

Ingredients:

- 1 teaspoon monk fruit
- 1 teaspoon almond butter
- 1 teaspoon coconut oil
- 2 tablespoons almonds, chopped
- 1 teaspoon pumpkin puree
- ½ teaspoon pumpkin pie spices
- 2 tablespoons coconut flakes
- 2 tablespoons pumpkin seeds, crushed
- 1 teaspoon hemp seeds
- 1 teaspoon flax seeds
- Cooking spray

Directions:

1.   In the big bowl mix up almond butter and coconut oil. Microwave the mixture until it is melted. After this, in the separated bowl mix up monk fruit, pumpkin spices, coconut flakes, pumpkin seeds, hemp seeds, and flax seeds. Add the melted coconut oil and pumpkin puree. Then stir the mixture until it is homogenous. Preheat the air fryer to 350F. Then put the pumpkin mixture on the baking paper and make the shape of the square.

2.   After this, cut the square on the serving bars and transfer in the preheated air fryer. Cook the pumpkin granola for 12 minutes.

Nutrition: calories 91, fat 8.2, fiber 1.4, carbs 3, protein 3

Pickled Bacon Bowls

Preparation time: 5 minutes

Prep time: 20 minutes

Servings: 4

Ingredients:

• 4 dill pickle spears, sliced in half and quartered 8 bacon slices, halved

• 1 cup avocado mayonnaise

Directions:

1. Wrap each pickle spear in a bacon slice, put them in your air fryer's basket and cook at 400 degrees F for 20 minutes. Divide into bowls and serve as a snack with the mayonnaise.

Nutrition: calories 100, fat 4, fiber 2, carbs 3, protein 4

Tomato Smokies

Prep time: 15 minutes

Prep time: 10 minutes

Servings: 10

Ingredients:

- 12 oz pork and beef smokies

- 3 oz bacon, sliced

- 1 teaspoon keto tomato sauce

- 1 teaspoon Erythritol

- 1 teaspoon avocado oil

- ½ teaspoon cayenne pepper

Directions:

1. Sprinkle the smokies with cayenne pepper and tomato sauce. Then sprinkle them with Erythritol and olive oil. After this, wrap every smokie in the bacon and secure it with the toothpick. Preheat the air fryer to 400F. Place the bacon smokies in the air fryer and cook them for 10 minutes.

2. Shake them gently during cooking to avoid burning.

Nutrition: calories 126, fat 9.7, fiber 0.1, carbs 1.4, protein 8.7

Coconut Chicken Bites

Preparation time: 5 minutes

Prep time: 20 minutes

Servings: 4

Ingredients:

- 2 teaspoons garlic powder 2 eggs

- Salt and black pepper to the taste

- ¾ cup coconut flakes Cooking spray

- pound chicken breasts, skinless, boneless and cubed

Directions:

1. Put the coconut in a bowl and mix the eggs with garlic powder, salt and pepper in a second one. Dredge the chicken cubes in eggs and then in coconut and arrange them all in your air fryer's basket. Grease with cooking spray, cook at 370 degrees F for 20 minutes. Arrange the chicken bites on a platter and serve as an appetizer.

Nutrition: calories 202, fat 12, fiber 2, carbs 4, protein 7

Pizza Bites

Prep time: 15 minutes

Prep time: 3 minutes

Servings: 10

Ingredients:

- 10 Mozzarella cheese slices
- 10 pepperoni slices

Directions:

1.   Preheat the air fryer to 400F. Line the air fryer pan with baking paper and put Mozzarella in it in one layer. After this, place the pan in the air fryer basket and cook the cheese for 3 minutes or until it is melted. After this, remove the cheese from the air fryer and cool it to room temperature.

2.   Then remove the melted cheese from the baking paper and put the pepperoni slices on it. Fold the cheese in the shape of turnovers.

Nutrition: calories 117, fat 10.4, fiber 0, carbs 0, protein 8.3

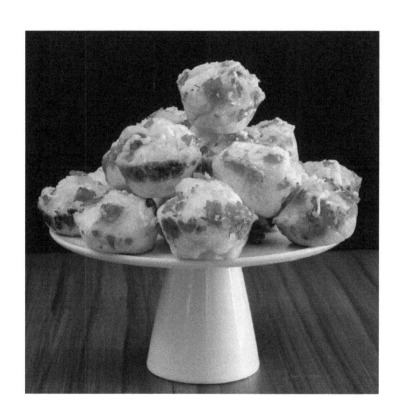

Mozzarella Snack

Preparation time: 5 minutes

Prep time: 5 minutes

Servings: 8

Ingredients:

- cups mozzarella, shredded

- ¾ cup almond flour

- 2 teaspoons psyllium husk powder

- ¼ teaspoon sweet paprika

Directions:

1.   Put the mozzarella in a bowl, melt it in the microwave for 2 minutes, add all the other ingredients quickly and stir really until you obtain a dough. Divide the dough into 2 balls, roll them on 2 baking sheets and cut into triangles. Arrange the tortillas in your air fryer's basket and bake at 370 degrees F for 5 minutes. Transfer to bowls and serve as a snack.

Nutrition: calories 170, fat 2, fiber 3, carbs 4, protein

Mushroom Pizza Bites

Prep time: 10 minutes

Prep time: 7 minutes

Servings: 6

Ingredients:

- 6 cremini mushroom caps

- 3 oz Parmesan, grated

- 1 tablespoon olive oil

- ½ tomato, chopped

- ½ teaspoon dried basil

- 1 teaspoon ricotta cheese

Directions:

1.   Preheat the air fryer to 400F. Sprinkle the mushroom caps with olive oil and put in the air fryer basket in one layer. Cook them for 3 minutes. After this, mix up tomato and ricotta cheese. Fill the mushroom

caps with tomato mixture. Then top them with parmesan and sprinkle with dried basil. Cook the mushroom pizzas for 4 minutes at 400F.

Nutrition: calories 73, fat 5.5, fiber 0.2, carbs 1.6, protein 5.2

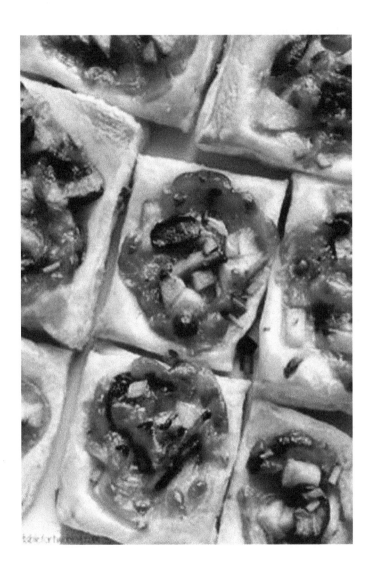

Paprika Chips

Preparation time: 2 minutes

Prep time: 5 minutes

Servings: 4

Ingredients:

- 8 ounces cheddar cheese, shredded 1 teaspoon sweet paprika

Directions:

1. Divide the cheese in small heaps in a pan that fits the air fryer, sprinkle the paprika on top, introduce the pan in the machine and cook at 400 degrees F for 5 minutes. Cool the chips down and serve them.

Nutrition: calories 150, fat 4, fiber 3, carbs 4, protein 6

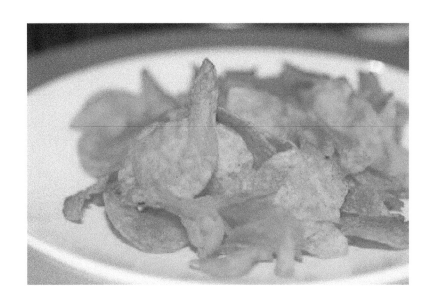

Lightning Source UK Ltd.
Milton Keynes UK
UKHW020634220621
385949UK00001B/55